Keto Vegetarian Cuisine

A Vegetarian Approach to a Healthy

Life Enhancing your Metabolism

Lauren Bellisario

Table of Contents

Gouda Breakfast Soufflés

Preparation time: 10minutes

Cooking time: 10minutes

Servings: 4

Nutritional Values (Per Serving):

- Calories: 570
- Total Fat: 57.6g
- Saturated Fat: 35.5g
- Total Carbs: 12 g
- Dietary Fiber: 5g
- Sugar: 3g
- Protein: 10g
- Sodium: 814mg

Ingredients:

- 2 ½ tbsp butter, softened
- 2 ½ tbsp almond flour
- 1 ½ tsp mustard powder
- ½ cup almond milk

- 2 ½ cup Gouda cheese, grated + a little extra for topping
- 4 yolks, beaten
- 2 egg whites, beaten until stiff

Directions:

1. Preheat the oven to 375 F and lightly brush the inner parts of four medium ramekins with ½ tablespoon of butter.
2. Melt the remaining 2 tablespoons of butter in a small pan over low heat and stir in the almond flour, cook for 1 minute, stirring constantly. Remove from the heat, mix in the mustard powder until evenly combined and slowly whisk in the milk until no lumps form.
3. Return to medium heat, while still stirring until the sauce comes to a rolling boil. Stir in the cheese until melted. Turn the heat off.
4. Into the egg yolks whisk ¼ cup of the warmed milk mixture, then combine with the remaining milk sauce. Fold in the egg whites gradually until evenly combined.
5. Spoon the mixture into the ramekins and top with the remaining cheese. Bake in the oven for 8 to 10 minutes or until the soufflés have a slight wobble, but soft at the center.
6. Allow cooling for 5 minutes and serve.

Raspberry, Hazelnut and Pecan Porridge

Preparation time: 8 minutes

Cooking time: 15 minutes

Serving: 2

Nutritional Values (Per Serving):

- Calories: 96
- Total Fat: 9.9g
- Saturated Fat:6.7 g
- Total Carbs: 2 g
- Dietary Fiber: 1
- Sugar: 1g
- Protein: 1g
- Sodium: 66mg

Ingredients:

- 2 tbsp coconut flour
- 1 tsp psyllium husk powder
- Salt to taste

- 6 tbsp coconut cream
- 2 oz butter
- 2 eggs
- 2 tbsp freshly squeezed lemon juice
- 1 tsp cinnamon powder
- 6 fresh raspberries, halved
- 4 tbsp chopped hazelnuts
- 2 tbsp chopped pecans

Directions:

1. In a medium saucepan, combine the coconut flour, psyllium husk powder, salt, coconut cream, egg, lemon juice, and cinnamon powder. Cook the Ingredients over low heat while stirring constantly but do not allow boiling until thickened.

2. Dish the porridge and top with the raspberries, hazelnuts, and pecans. Serve warm.

Tempeh Coconut Curry Bake

Preparation time: 7 minutes

Cooking time: 23 minutes

Serving: 4

Nutritional Values (Per Serving):

- Calories:417
- Total Fat:38.8g
- Saturated Fat:22.4g
- Total Carbs: 11g
- Dietary Fiber:2g
- Sugar: 3g
- Protein: 11g
- Sodium: 194mg

Ingredients:

- 1 oz. plant butter, for greasing

- 2 ½ cups chopped tempeh
- Salt and black pepper
- 4 tbsp plant butter
- 2 tbsp red curry paste
- 1 ½ cup coconut cream
- ½ cup fresh parsley, chopped
- 15 oz. cauliflower, cut into florets

Directions:

1. Preheat the oven to 400 F and grease a baking dish with 1 ounce of butter.
2. Arrange the tempeh in the baking dish, sprinkle with salt and black pepper, and top each tempeh with a slice of the remaining butter.
3. In a bowl, mix the red curry paste with the coconut cream and parsley. Pour the mixture over the tempeh.
4. Bake in the oven for 20 minutes or until the tempeh is cooked.
5. While baking, season the cauliflower with salt, place in a microwave-safe bowl, and sprinkle with some water. Steam in the microwave for 3 minutes or until the cauliflower is soft and tender within.
6. Remove the curry bake and serve with the caulis.

Kale and Mushroom Pierogis

Prep Time:15 minutes

Cooking time: 30 minutes

Serving: 4

Nutritional Values (Per Serving):

- Calories:364
- Total Fat:33.4 g
- Saturated Fat:17.3 g
- Total Carbs:8g
- Dietary Fiber:2g
- Sugar:3 g
- Protein:12 g
- Sodium:779 mg

Ingredients:

For the stuffing:

- 2 tbsp butter
- 2 garlic cloves, finely chopped

- 1 small red onion, finely chopped
- 3 oz. baby bella mushrooms, sliced
- 2 oz. fresh kale
- ½ tsp salt
- ¼ tsp black pepper
- ½ cup cashew cream
- 2 oz. grated tofu cheese

For the pierogi:

- 1 tbsp flax seed powder + 3 tbsp water
- ½ cup almond flour
- 4 tbsp coconut flour
- ½ tsp salt
- 1 tsp baking powder
- 1½ cups shredded tofu cheese
- 5 tbsp butter
- Olive oil for brushing

Directions:

1. Put the butter in a skillet and melt over medium heat, then add and sauté the garlic, red onion, mushrooms, and kale until the mushrooms brown.

2. Season the mixture with salt and black pepper and reduce the heat to low. Stir in the cashew cream and tofu cheese and simmer for 1 minute. Turn the heat off and set the filling aside to cool.

3. Make the pierogis: In a small bowl, mix the flax seed powder with water and allow sitting for 5 minutes.

4. In a bowl, combine the almond flour, coconut flour, salt, and baking powder.

5. Put a small pan over low heat, add, and melt the tofu cheese and butter while stirring continuously until smooth batter forms. Turn the heat off.

6. Pour the flax egg into the cream mixture, continue stirring, while adding the flour mixture until a firm dough forms.

7. Mold the dough into four balls, place on a chopping board, and use a rolling pin to flatten each into ½ inch thin round pieces.

8. Spread a generous amount of stuffing on one-half of each dough, then fold over the filling, and seal the dough with your fingers.

9. Brush with olive oil, place on a baking sheet, and bake for 20 minutes or until the pierogis turn a golden brown color.

10. Serve the pierogis with a lettuce tomato salad.

Mushroom Lettuce Wraps

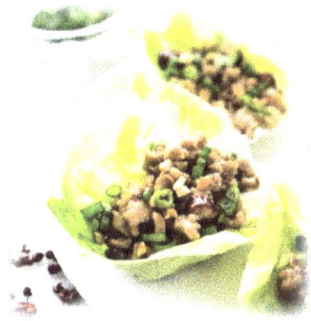

Preparation time: 5minutes

Cooking time: 16minutes

 Serving: 4

Nutritional Values (Per Serving):

- Calories:439
- Total Fat:31.9 g
- Saturated Fat:12.2 g
- Total Carbs: 9 g
- Dietary Fiber:4g
- Sugar:1 g
- Protein:36g
- Sodium: 574mg

Ingredients:

- 2 tbsp butter
- 4 oz. baby bella mushrooms, sliced
- 1½ lbs. tofu, crumbled
- ½ tsp salt
- ¼ tsp black pepper
- 1 iceberg lettuce, leaves extracted
- 1 cup shredded cheddar cheese
- 1 large tomato, sliced

Directions:

1. Put the butter in a skillet and melt over medium heat. Add the mushrooms and sauté until browned and tender, about 6 minutes. Transfer the mushrooms to a plate and set aside.
2. Add the tofu to the skillet, season with salt and black pepper, and cook until brown, about 10 minutes. Turn the heat off.
3. Spoon the tofu and mushrooms into the lettuce leaves, sprinkle with the cheddar cheese, and share the tomato slices on top.
4. Serve the burger immediately.

Green Avocado Carbonara

Preparation time: 15minutes

Cooking time: 15minutes

Serving: 4

Nutritional Values (Per Serving):

- Calories:941
- Total Fat:94.2g
- Saturated Fat:30.4g
- Total Carbs:19g
- Dietary Fiber:8g
- Sugar:5g
- Protein:16g
- Sodium:1314mg

Ingredients:

- 8 tbsp flax seed powder + 1 ½ cups water
- 1 ½ cups dairy-free cashew cream

- 1 tsp salt
- 5 ½ tbsp psyllium husk powder

Avocado sauce

- 1 avocado, peeled and pitted
- 1 ¾ cups coconut cream
- Juice of ½ lemon
- 1 teaspoon onion powder
- ½ teaspoon garlic powder
- ¼ cup olive oil
- ¾ teaspoon sea salt
- ¼ teaspoon black pepper
- Walnut Parmesan or store-bought parmesan

For serving

- 4 tbsp toasted pecans
- ½ cup freshly grated tofu cheese

Directions:

1. Preheat the oven to 300 F.
2. In a medium bowl, mix the flax seed powder with water and allow sitting to thicken for 5 minutes.

3. Add the cashew cream, salt, and psyllium husk powder. Whisk until smooth batter forms.

4. Line a baking sheet with parchment paper, pour in the batter and cover with another parchment paper. Use a rolling pin to flatten the dough into the sheet.

5. Place in the oven and bake for 10 to 12 minutes. Remove the pasta after, take off the parchment papers and use a sharp knife to slice the pasta into thin strips lengthwise. Cut each piece into halves, pour into a bowl, and set aside.

6. For the avocado sauce, in a blender, combine the avocado, coconut cream, lemon juice, onion powder, and garlic powder. Puree the Ingredients until smooth.

7. Pour the olive oil over the pasta and stir to coat properly. Pour the avocado sauce on top and mix. Then, season with salt, black pepper, and the soy cheese. Combine again.

8. Divide the pasta into serving plates, garnish with extra soy cheese and pecans, and serve immediately.

Cashew Buttered Quesadillas with Leafy Greens

Preparation time: 10minutes

Cooking time: 20minutes

Serving: 4

Nutritional Values (Per Serving):

- Calories:224
- Total Fat:20.4g
- Saturated Fat:12.2g
- Total Carbs: 1g
- Dietary Fiber:0g
- Sugar:1g
- Protein:9g
- Sodium:556mg

Ingredients:

Tortillas

- 3 tbsp flax seed powder + ½ cup water
- ½ cup dairy-free cashew cream
- 1½ tsp psyllium husk powder
- 1 tbsp coconut flour
- ½ tsp salt

Filling

- 1 tbsp cashew butter, for frying
- 5 oz. grated cheddar cheese
- 1 oz. leafy greens

Directions:

1. Preheat the oven to 400 F.
2. In a bowl, mix the flax seed powder with water and allow sitting to thicken for 5 minutes.
3. After, whisk the cashew cream into the flax egg until the batter is smooth.
4. In another bowl, combine the psyllium husk powder, coconut flour, and salt. Add the flour mixture to the flax

egg batter and fold in until fully incorporated. Allow sitting for a few minutes.

5. Then, line a baking sheet with parchment paper and pour in the mixture. Spread into the baking sheet using a spatula and bake in the upper rack of the oven for 5 to 7 minutes or until brown around the edges. Keep a watchful eye on the tortillas to prevent burning.

6. Remove when ready and slice into 8 pieces. Set aside.

7. For the filling, spoon a little cashew butter into a skillet and place a tortilla in the pan. Sprinkle with some cheddar cheese, leafy greens, and cover with another tortilla.

8. Brown each side of the quesadilla for 1 minute or until the cheese melts. Transfer to a plate.

9. Repeat assembling the quesadillas using the remaining cashew butter.

10. Serve immediately with avocado salad.

Zucchini Boats with Cheese

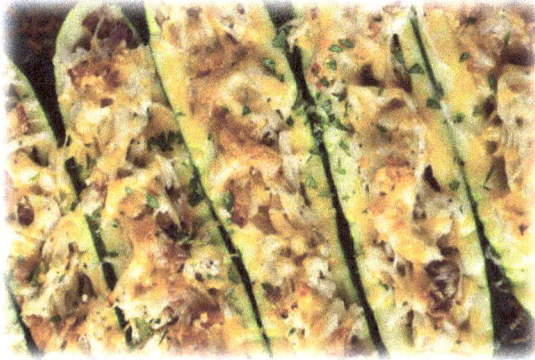

Preparation time: 3minutes

Cooking time: 4minutes

Serving: 2

Nutritional Values (Per Serving):

- Calories:721
- Total Fat:76.8g
- Saturated Fat:21.2g
- Total Carbs: 2g
- Dietary Fiber:0g
- Sugar:0g

- Protein:9g
- Sodium:309mg

Ingredients:

- 1 medium-sized zucchini
- 4 tbsp butter
- 2 garlic cloves, minced
- 1½ oz. baby kale
- Salt and black pepper to taste
- 2 tbsp unsweetened tomato sauce
- 1 cup cheese
- Olive oil for drizzling

Directions:

1. Preheat the oven to 375 F.
2. Use a knife to slice the zucchini in halves and scoop out the pulp with a spoon into a plate. Keep the flesh.
3. Grease a baking sheet with cooking spray and place the zucchini boats on top.

4. Put the butter in a skillet and melt over medium heat. Add and sauté the garlic until fragrant and slightly browned, about 4 minutes.

5. Add the kale and the zucchini pulp. Cook until the kale wilts; season with salt and black pepper.

6. Spoon the tomato sauce into the boats and spread to coat the bottom evenly. Then, spoon the kale mixture into the zucchinis and sprinkle with the cheese.

7. Bake in the oven for 20 to 25 minutes or until the cheese has a beautiful golden color.

8. Plate the zucchinis when ready, drizzle with olive oil, and season with salt and black pepper.

9. Serve immediately.

Tempeh Garam Masala Bake

Preparation time: 5minutes

Cooking time: 24minutes

Serving: 4

Nutritional Values (Per Serving):

- Calories:286
- Total Fat:27g
- Saturated Fat:15g
- Total Carbs: 5g
- Dietary Fiber:0g
- Sugar:1g
- Protein:9g
- Sodium:87mg

Ingredients:

- 3 tbsp butter
- 3 cups tempeh slices

- Salt
- 2 tbsp garam masala
- 1 green bell pepper, finely diced
- 1¼ cups coconut cream
- 1 tbsp fresh cilantro, finely chopped

Directions:

1. Preheat the oven to 400 F.
2. Place a skillet over medium heat, add, and melt the butter. Meanwhile, season the tempeh with some salt. Fry the tempeh in the butter until browned on both sides, about 4 minutes.
3. Stir half of the garam masala into the tempeh until evenly mixed; turn the heat off.
4. Transfer the tempeh with the spice into a baking dish.
5. Then, in a small bowl, mix the green bell pepper, coconut cream, cilantro, and remaining garam masala.
6. Pour the mixture over the tempeh and bake in the oven for 20 minutes or until golden brown on top.
7. Garnish with cilantro and serve with some cauli rice.

Caprese Casserole

Preparation time: 5minutes

Cooking time: 20minutes

Serving: 4

Nutritional Values (Per Serving):

- Calories:588
- Total Fat:59g
- Saturated Fat:11g
- Total Carbs: 2g
- Dietary Fiber:1g
- Sugar:1g
- Protein:13g
- Sodium: 646mg

Ingredients:

- 1 cup cherry tomatoes, halved
- 1 cup mozzarella cheese, cut into small pieces

- 2 tbsp basil pesto
- 1 cup vegan mayonnaise
- 2 oz. tofu cheese
- Salt and black pepper
- 1 cup arugula
- 4 tbsp olive oil

Directions:

1. Preheat the oven to 350 F.
2. In a baking dish, mix the cherry tomatoes, mozzarella, basil pesto, mayonnaise, half of the tofu cheese, salt, and black pepper.
3. Level the Ingredients with a spatula and sprinkle the remaining tofu cheese on top. Bake for 20 minutes or until the top of the casserole is golden brown.
4. Remove and allow cooling for a few minutes. Slice and dish into plates, top with some arugula and drizzle with olive oil. Serve.

Herb Baby Potatoes

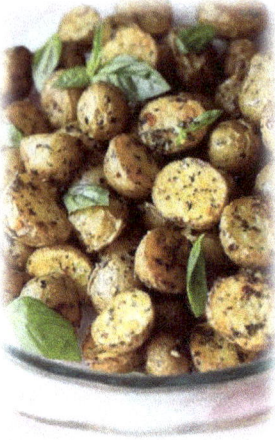

Preparation time: 10 minutes

Cooking time: 25 minutes

Servings: 2

Nutritional Values (per Serving):

- Calories 125
- Fat 0.2 g

- Carbohydrates 27.3 g
- Sugar 2.1 g
- Protein 3 g
- Cholesterol 0 mg

Ingredients:

- 1 lb potatoes, cut into 1-inch pieces
- 1/4 tsp dried basil
- 1/4 tsp pepper
- 1/4 tsp dried oregano
- 1/4 tsp salt

Directions:

1. Preheat the air fryer to 400 F.
2. Add potatoes, basil, oregano, pepper, and salt in a bowl and toss well.
3. Transfer potatoes into the air fryer basket and cook for 25 minutes. Stir halfway through.
4. Serve and enjoy.

Nutritious Broccoli

Preparation time: 10 minutes

Cooking time: 20 minutes

Servings: 2

Nutritional Values (per Serving):

- Calories 130
- Fat 9.7 g
- Carbohydrates 8.9 g
- Sugar 2 g
- Protein 4.3 g
- Cholesterol 0 mg

Ingredients:

- 1/2 lb broccoli florets
- 1 tbsp walnuts, chopped
- 1 tbsp olive oil
- 1 tbsp vinegar

- Pepper
- Salt

Directions:

1. Preheat the air fryer to 360 F.
2. Add all ingredients into the bowl and toss well. Add broccoli mixture into the air fryer basket and cook for 20 minutes. Stir halfway through.
3. Serve and enjoy.

Spicy Brussels Sprouts

Preparation time: 10 minutes

Cooking time: 14 minutes

Servings: 2

Nutritional Values (per Serving):

- Calories 85
- Fat 4.1 g
- Carbohydrates 11 g
- Sugar 2.6 g
- Protein 4.1 g
- Cholesterol 0 mg

Ingredients:

- 1/2 lb Brussels sprouts, trimmed and halved
- 1/2 tsp cayenne
- 1/2 tbsp olive oil

- Pepper
- Salt

Directions:

1. Preheat the air fryer to 370 F.
2. Add all ingredients into the bowl and toss well.
3. Add Brussels sprouts mixture into the air fryer basket and cook for 14 minutes. Stir halfway through.
4. Serve and enjoy.

Lime Olive Potatoes

Preparation time: 10 minutes

Cooking time: 20 minutes

Servings: 2

Nutritional Values (per Serving):

- Calories 275
- Fat 11.1 g
- Carbohydrates 42.2 g
- Sugar 4.2 g
- Protein 4.7 g
- Cholesterol 0 mg

Ingredients:

- 1 lb potatoes, peeled and cubed
- 1/2 cup olives, pitted and halved
- 1 tbsp olive oil
- 1/2 tbsp lime juice

- ¼ tsp chili powder
- 1/2 onion, sliced
- Pepper
- Salt

Directions:

1. Preheat the air fryer to 400 F.
2. Add all ingredients into the bowl and toss well.
3. Add potato olive mixture into the air fryer basket and cook for 20 minutes. Stir halfway through.
4. Serve and enjoy.

Tasty Baby Carrots

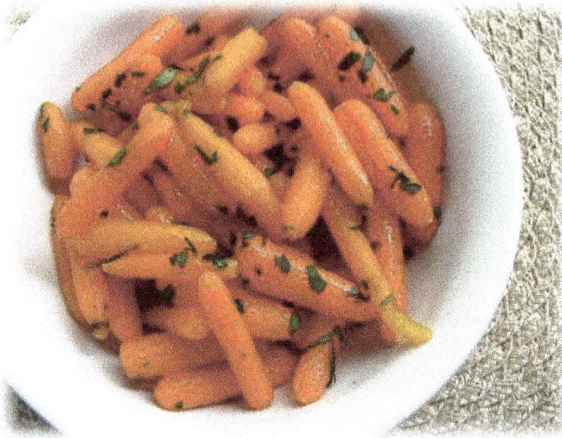

Preparation time: 10 minutes

Cooking time: 20 minutes

Servings: 2

Nutritional Values (per Serving):

- Calories 120
- Fat 8.9 g
- Carbohydrates 10 g
- Sugar 5.4 g

- Protein 0.9 g
- Cholesterol 23 mg

Ingredients:

- 1/2 lb baby carrots, peeled
- ¼ tsp cinnamon
- 1 1/2 tbsp butter, melted
- Pepper
- Salt

Directions:

1. Preheat the air fryer to 380 F.
2. Add all ingredients into the bowl and toss well.
3. Add baby carrots into the air fryer basket and cook for 20 minutes. Stir halfway through.
4. Serve and enjoy.

Cherry Tomato & Green Beans

Preparation time: 10 minutes

Cooking time: 15 minutes

Servings: 2

Nutritional Values (per Serving):

- Calories 142
- Fat 9.6 g
- Carbohydrates 10.3 g
- Sugar 2.8 g
- Protein 6.1 g
- Cholesterol 8 mg

Ingredients:

- 1/2 lb green beans, trimmed
- 1/4 cup parmesan cheese, shredded
- 1 tbsp butter, melted
- 1/2 cup cherry tomatoes, halved

- Pepper
- Salt

Directions:

1. Preheat the air fryer to 375 F.
2. In a bowl, toss green beans, cherry tomatoes, butter, pepper, and salt.
3. Add green beans and tomato mixture into the air fryer basket and cook for 15 minutes.
4. Sprinkle with cheese and serve.

Green Salad

Preparation time: 10 minutes

Cooking time: 0 minutes

Servings: 4

Nutritional Values (Per Serving):

- Calories – 120
- Fat – 2
- Fiber – 1
- Carbs – 4
- Protein - 5

Ingredients:

- 24 green grapes, halved
- 1 bunch Swiss chard, chopped
- 1 avocado, pitted, peeled, and cubed

- Salt and ground black pepper, to taste
- 2 tablespoons avocado oil
- 1 tablespoon mustard
- 7 sage leaves, chopped
- 1 garlic clove, peeled and minced

Directions:

1. In a salad bowl, mix the Swiss chard with the grapes and avocado cubes.
2. In a bowl, mix the mustard with the oil, sage, garlic, salt, and pepper, and whisk.
3. Add this to the salad, toss to coat well, and serve.

Catalan-style Greens

Preparation time: 10 minutes

Cooking time: 15 minutes

Servings: 4

Nutritional Values (Per Serving):

- Calories – 120
- Fat – 1
- Fiber – 2
- Carbs – 3
- Protein - 6

Ingredients:

- 1 apple, cored and chopped
- 1 onion, peeled and sliced
- 3 tablespoons avocado oil
- ¼ cup raisins
- 6 garlic cloves, peeled and chopped

- ¼ cup pine nuts, toasted
- ¼ cup balsamic vinegar
- 2½ cups Swiss chard
- 2½ cups spinach
- Salt and ground black pepper, to taste
- A pinch of nutmeg

Directions:

1. Heat up a pan with the oil over medium-high heat, add the onion, stir, and cook for 3 minutes.
2. Add the apple, stir, and cook for 4 minutes.
3. Add the garlic, stir, and cook for 1 minute.
4. Add the raisins, vinegar, spinach, and chard, stir, and cook for 5 minutes.
5. Add the nutmeg, salt, and pepper, stir, cook for a few seconds, divide on plates, and serve.

Swiss Chard and Chicken Soup

Preparation time: 10 minutes

Cooking time: 35 minutes

Servings: 12

Nutritional Values (Per Serving):

- Calories – 140
- Fat – 4
- Fiber – 2
- Carbs – 4
- Protein - 18

Ingredients:

- 4 cups Swiss chard, chopped
- 4 cups chicken breast, cooked, and shredded
- 2 cups water
- 1 cup mushrooms, sliced
- 1 tablespoon garlic, minced

- 1 tablespoon coconut oil, melted
- ¼ cup onion, peeled and chopped
- 8 cups chicken stock
- 2 cups yellow squash, chopped
- 1 cup green beans, cut into medium-sized pieces
- 2 tablespoons vinegar
- ¼ cup fresh basil, chopped
- Salt and ground black pepper, to taste
- 4 bacon slices, chopped
- ¼ cup sundried tomatoes, cored and chopped

Directions:

1. Heat up a pot with the oil over medium-high heat, add the bacon, stir, and cook for 2 minutes.
2. Add the tomatoes, garlic, onions, and mushrooms, stir, and cook for 5 minutes.
3. Add the water, stock, and chicken, stir, and cook for 15 minutes.
4. Add the Swiss chard, green beans, squash, salt, and pepper, stir, and cook for 10 minutes.
5. Add the vinegar, basil, salt, and pepper, stir, ladle into soup bowls, and serve.

Roasted Tomato Cream

Preparation time: 10 minutes

Cooking time: 1 hour

Servings: 8

Nutritional Values (Per Serving):

- Calories – 140
- Fat – 2
- Fiber – 2
- Carbs – 5
- Protein - 8

Ingredients:

- 1 jalapeño pepper, chopped
- 4 garlic cloves, peeled and minced
- 2 pounds cherry tomatoes, cut in half
- 1 onion, peeled and cut into wedges
- Salt and ground black pepper, to taste

- ¼ cup olive oil
- ½ teaspoon dried oregano
- 4 cups chicken stock
- ¼ cup fresh basil, chopped
- ½ cup Parmesan cheese, grated

Directions:

1. Spread the tomatoes, and onion in a baking dish.
2. Add the garlic and chili pepper, season with salt, pepper, and oregano, and drizzle the oil.
3. Toss to coat and bake in the oven at 425°F for 30 minutes.
4. Take the tomato mixture out of the oven, transfer to a pot, add the stock, and heat everything up over medium-high heat.
5. Bring to a boil, cover the pot, reduce heat, and simmer for 20 minutes.
6. Blend using an immersion blender, add the salt and pepper to taste, and basil, stir, and ladle into soup bowls. Sprinkle with Parmesan cheese on top and serve.

Eggplant Soup

Preparation time: 10 minutes

Cooking time: 50 minutes

Servings: 4

Nutritional Values (Per Serving):

- Calories – 180
- Fat – 2
- Fiber – 3
- Carbs – 5
- Protein - 10

Ingredients:

- 4 tomatoes
- 1 teaspoon garlic, minced
- ¼ onion, peeled and chopped
- Salt and ground black pepper, to taste
- 2 cups chicken stock

- 1 bay leaf
- ½ cup heavy cream
- 2 tablespoons fresh basil, chopped
- 4 tablespoons Parmesan cheese, grated
- 1 tablespoon olive oil
- 1 eggplant, chopped

Directions:

1. Spread the eggplant pieces on a baking sheet, mix with oil, onion, garlic, salt, and pepper, place in an oven at 400°F, and bake for 15 minutes.
2. Put water in a pot, bring to a boil over medium heat, add the tomatoes, steam them for 1 minute, peel them, and chop.
3. Take the eggplant mixture out of the oven, and transfer to a pot.
4. Add the tomatoes, stock, bay leaf, salt, and pepper, stir, bring to a boil, and simmer for 30 minutes.
5. Add the heavy cream, basil, and Parmesan cheese, stir, ladle into soup bowls, and serve.

Eggplant Stew

Preparation time: 10 minutes

Cooking time: 30 minutes

 Servings: 4

Nutritional Values (Per Serving):

- Calories – 200
- Fat – 13
- Fiber – 3
- Carbs – 5
- Protein - 7

Ingredients:

- 1 onion, peeled and chopped
- 2 garlic cloves, peeled and chopped
- 1 bunch fresh parsley, chopped
- Salt and ground black pepper, to taste
- 1 teaspoon dried oregano

- 2 eggplants, cut into medium-sized chunks
- 2 tablespoons olive oil
- 2 tablespoons capers, chopped
- 12 green olives, pitted and sliced
- 5 tomatoes, cored and chopped
- 3 tablespoons herb vinegar

Directions:

1. Heat up a pot with the oil over medium heat, add the eggplant, oregano, salt, and pepper, stir, and cook for 5 minutes.
2. Add the garlic, onion, and parsley, stir, and cook for 4 minutes.
3. Add the capers, olives, vinegar, and tomatoes, stir, and cook for 15 minutes.
4. Add more salt and pepper, if needed, stir, divide into bowls, and serve.

Black and Gold Gazpacho

Preparation time: 15 Minutes

Cooking time: 0 Minutes

Servings: 4

Ingredients:

- 1½ pounds ripe yellow tomatoes, chopped
- 1 large cucumber, peeled, seeded, and chopped
- 1 large yellow bell pepper, seeded, and chopped
- 4 green onions, white part only
- 2 garlic cloves, minced
- 2 tablespoons olive oil
- 2 tablespoons white wine vinegar
- Salt
- Ground cayenne
- 1½ cups cooked or 1 (15.5-ounce) can black beans, drained and rinsed

- 2 tablespoons minced fresh parsley
- 1 cup toasted croutons (optional)

Directions:

1. In a blender or food processor, combine half the tomatoes with the cucumber, bell pepper, green onions, and garlic. Process until smooth. Add the oil and vinegar, season with salt and cayenne to taste, and process until blended.
2. Transfer the soup to a large nonmetallic bowl and stir in the black beans and remaining tomatoes. Cover the bowl and refrigerate for 1 to 2 hours. Taste, adjusting seasonings if necessary.
3. Ladle the soup into bowls, garnish with parsley and croutons, if using, and serve.

Black-Eyed Pea & Sweet Potato Soup

Preparation time: 10 Minutes

Cooking time: 25 Minutes

Servings: 4

Nutrition per Serving (2 cups):

- Calories: 224
- Protein: 9g
- Total fat: 2g
- Saturated fat: 0g
- Carbohydrates: 46g
- Fiber: 10g

Ingredients:

- 1 teaspoon olive oil
- 2 to 3 cups peeled, cubed sweet potato, squash, or pumpkin
- ½ onion, chopped

- 1 garlic clove, minced Salt
- 2 cups water
- 1 (15-ounce) can black-eyed peas, drained and rinsed
- 2 tablespoons freshly squeezed lime juice
- 1 tablespoon sugar
- 1 teaspoon smoked or regular paprika
- Pinch red pepper flakes or cayenne pepper
- 3 cups shredded cabbage
- 1 cup corn kernels, thawed if frozen, drained if canned

Directions:

1. Heat the olive oil in a large soup pot over medium-high heat.
2. Add the sweet potato, onion, garlic, and a pinch of salt. Sauté for 3 to 4 minutes, until the onion and garlic are softened. Add the water, black-eyed peas, lime juice, sugar, paprika, red pepper flakes, and salt to taste. Bring to a boil and cook for 15 minutes. Add the cabbage and corn to the pot, stirring to combine, and cook for 5 minutes more, or until the sweet potato is tender.
3. Turn off the heat, let cool for a few minutes, and serve. Leftovers will keep in an airtight container for up to 1 week in the refrigerator or up to 1 month in the freezer.

Soba and Green Lentil Soup

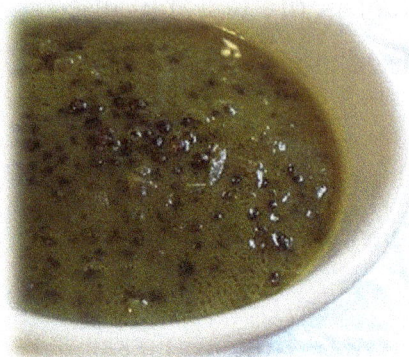

Preparation time: 5 Minutes

Cooking time: 55 Minutes

Servings: 4 To 6

Ingredients:

- 2 tablespoons olive oil
- 1 medium onion, minced
- 1 medium carrot, halved lengthwise and sliced diagonally
- 2 garlic cloves, minced
- 1 (28-ounce) can crushed tomatoes

- 1 cup green (French) lentils, picked over, rinsed, and drained
- 1 teaspoon dried thyme
- 6 cups vegetable broth, (homemade, store-bought or water)
- Salt and freshly ground black pepper
- 4 ounces soba noodles, broken into thirds

Directions:

1. In a large soup pot over medium heat, heat the oil. Add the onion, carrot, and garlic. Cover and cook until softened, about 7 minutes. Uncover and stir in the tomatoes, lentils, thyme, and broth and bring to a boil. Reduce heat to medium, season with salt and pepper to taste, and cover and simmer until the lentils are just tender, about 45 minutes.
2. Stir in the noodles and cook until tender, about 10 minutes longer, and serve.

Lemongrass Tempeh with Spaghetti Squash

Preparation time: 1 hour + 45 minutes marinating time

Serving size: 4

Nutritional Values (Per Serving):

- Calories:457
- Total Fat:37g
- Saturated Fat:8.1g
- Total Carbs:17g
- Dietary Fiber:5g
- Sugar:4g
- Protein:22g
- Sodium:656mg

Ingredients:

For the lemongrass tempeh:

- 2 tbsp minced lemongrass
- 2 tbsp fresh ginger paste
- 2 tbsp sugar-free maple syrup
- 2 tbsp coconut aminos
- 1 tbsp Himalayan salt
- 4 tempeh
- 2 tbsp avocado oil

For the squash noodles:

- 3 lb spaghetti squashes, halved and deseeded
- 1 tbsp olive oil
- Salt and black pepper to taste

For the steamed spinach:

- 1 tbsp avocado oil
- 1 tsp fresh ginger paste
- 1 lb baby spinach

For the peanut-coconut sauce:

- ½ cup coconut milk
- ¼ cup organic almond butter

Directions:

1. In a medium bowl, mix the lemongrass, ginger paste, maple syrup, coconut aminos, and Himalayan salt. Place the tempeh in the liquid and coat well. Allow marinating for 45 minutes.
2. After, heat the avocado oil in a large skillet, remove the tempeh from the marinade and sear in the oil on both sides until golden brown and cooked through, 10 to 15 minutes. Transfer to a plate and cover with foil.

For the spaghetti squash:

3. Preheat the oven to 380 F.
4. Place the spaghetti squashes on a baking sheet, brush with the olive oil and season with salt and black pepper. Bake in the oven for 20 to 25 minutes or until tender.
5. When ready, remove the squash and shred with two forks into spaghetti-like strands. Keep warm in the oven.

For the spinach:

6. In another skillet, heat the avocado oil and sauté the ginger until fragrant. Add the spinach and cook to wilt while stirring to be coated well in the ginger, 2 minutes. Turn the heat off.

For the almond-coconut sauce:

7. In a medium bowl, quickly whisk the coconut milk with the almond butter until well combined.

To serve:

8. Unwrap and divide the tempeh into four bowls, add the spaghetti squash to the side, then the spinach and drizzle the almond sauce on top.
9. Serve immediately.

Caesar Salad

Preparation time: 10 Minutes

Cooking time: 0 Minutes

Servings: 1

Nutrition per Serving (in a meal):

- Calories: 415
- Protein: 19g
- Total fat: 8g
- Saturated fat: 1g
- Carbohydrates: 72g
- Fiber: 13g

Ingredients:

For The Caesar Salad

- 2 cups chopped romaine lettuce
- 2 tablespoons Caesar Dressing
- 1 serving Herbed Croutons or store-bought croutons
- Vegan cheese, grated (optional)

Make It a Meal

- ½ cup cooked pasta
- ½ cup canned chickpeas, drained and rinsed
- 2 additional tablespoons Caesar Dressing

Directions:

For the Caesar Salad

1. In a large bowl, toss together the lettuce, dressing, croutons, and cheese (if using).

To Make It a Meal

2. Add the pasta, chickpeas, and additional dressing. Toss to coat.

Classic Potato Salad

Preparation time: 10 Minutes

Cooking time: 15 Minutes

Servings: 4

Nutrition per Serving:

- Calories: 269
- Protein: 6g
- Total fat: 5g
- Saturated fat: 1g
- Carbohydrates: 51g
- Fiber: 6g

Ingredients:

- 6 potatoes, scrubbed or peeled and chopped
- Pinch salt
- ½ cup Creamy Tahini Dressing or vegan mayo
- 1 teaspoon dried dill (optional)

- 1 teaspoon Dijon mustard (optional)
- 4 celery stalks, chopped
- 2 scallions, white and light green parts only, chopped

Directions:

1. Put the potatoes in a large pot, add the salt, and pour in enough water to cover. Bring the water to a boil over high heat. Cook the potatoes for 15 to 20 minutes, until soft. Drain and set aside to cool. (Alternatively, put the potatoes in a large microwave-safe dish with a bit of water. Cover and heat on high power for 10 minutes.)

2. In a large bowl, whisk together the dressing, dill (if using), and mustard (if using). Toss the celery and scallions with the dressing. Add the cooked, cooled potatoes and toss to combine. Store leftovers in an airtight container in the refrigerator for up to 1 week.

Brown Rice and Pepper Salad

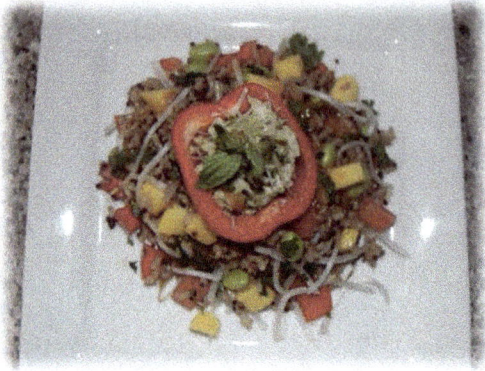

Preparation time: 15 Minutes

Cooking time: 0 Minutes

Servings: 4

Ingredients:

- 2 cups prepared brown rice
- ½ red onion, diced
- 1 red bell pepper, diced
- 2 tablespoons unseasoned rice vinegar
- 1 tablespoon soy sauce
- 1 garlic clove, minced

- 1 tablespoon grated fresh ginger
- ¼ teaspoon sea salt
- ¼ teaspoon freshly ground black pepper
- 1 orange bell pepper, diced
- 1 carrot, diced
- ¼ cup olive oil

Directions:

1. In a large bowl, combine the rice, onion, bell peppers, and carrot. In a small bowl, whisk together the olive oil, rice vinegar, soy sauce, garlic, ginger, salt, and pepper. Toss with the rice mixture and serve immediately.

Mediterranean Orzo & Chickpea Salad

Preparation time: 15 Minutes

Cooking time: 8 Minutes

Servings: 4

Nutrition per Serving:

- Calories: 233
- Protein: 6g
- Total fat: 15g
- Saturated fat: 2g
- Carbohydrates: 20g
- Fiber: 5g

Ingredients:

- ¼ cup olive oil
- 2 tablespoons freshly squeezed lemon juice

- Pinch salt
- 1½ cups canned chickpeas, drained and rinsed
- 2 cups orzo or other small pasta shape, cooked according to the package directions: drained, and rinsed with cold water to cool
- 2 cups raw spinach, finely chopped
- 1 cup chopped cucumber
- ¼ red onion, finely diced

Directions:

1. In a large bowl, whisk together the olive oil, lemon juice, and salt. Add the chickpeas and cooked orzo, and toss to coat.
2. Stir in the spinach, cucumber, and red onion. Store leftovers in an airtight container in the refrigerator for up to 5 days.

Easy Banana Chips

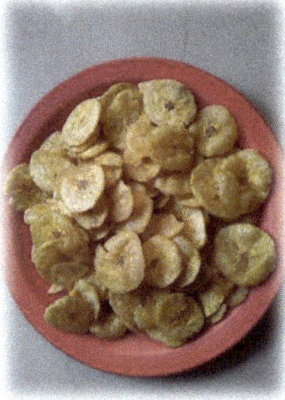

Preparation time: 10 minutes

Cooking time: 15 minutes

Servings: 2

Nutritional Values (per Serving):

- Calories 84
- Fat 2.7 g
- Carbohydrates 16.1 g
- Sugar 8.4 g

- Protein 0.8 g
- Cholesterol 0 mg

Ingredients:

- 1 large raw bananas, peel and sliced
- 1/4 tsp turmeric powder
- 1 tsp olive oil
- 1 tsp salt

Directions:

1. In a bowl add water, turmeric powder, and salt. Stir well.
2. Add sliced bananas in bowl water soak for 10 minutes. Drain well and pat dry chips with a paper towel.
3. Add banana slices to a bowl and toss with oil and salt.
4. Place banana slices into the air fryer basket and cook at 350 F for 15 minutes. Turn halfway through.
5. Serve and enjoy.

Sweet Potato Bites

Preparation time: 10 minutes

Cooking time: 15 minutes

Servings: 2

Nutritional Values (per Serving):

- Calories 301
- Fat 14.3 g
- Carbohydrates 43.2 g
- Sugar 24.8 g
- Protein 2.9 g
- Cholesterol 0 mg

Ingredients:

- 2 sweet potato, diced into 1-inch cubes
- 2 tbsp olive oil
- 2 tbsp honey
- 1 1/2 tsp cinnamon

Directions:

1. Preheat the air fryer to 350 F.
2. Add all ingredients into the bowl and toss well.
3. Add sweet potato into the air fryer basket and cook for 15 minutes.
4. Serve and enjoy.

Fish Nuggets

Preparation time: 10 minutes

Cooking time: 10 minutes

Servings: 4

Nutritional Values (per Serving):

- Calories 497
- Fat 18.6 g
- Carbohydrates 44.1 g
- Sugar 2.2 g
- Protein 37 g
- Cholesterol 185 mg

Ingredients:

- 3 eggs, lightly beaten
- 1 lb cod fish fillet, cut into chunks
- 1/4 cup olive oil
- 1 cup all-purpose flour

- 1 tsp garlic powder
- 1 cup breadcrumbs
- 1/4 tsp pepper
- 1 tsp salt

Directions:

1. Preheat the air fryer to 400 F.
2. In a small bowl, add eggs and whisk well.
3. In a separate bowl, add flour.
4. In a shallow dish, mix together breadcrumbs, garlic powder, pepper, salt, and oil.
5. Dip fish chunks into the egg then roll in flour and coat with breadcrumb mixture.
6. Place coated nuggets into the air fryer basket and cook at 400 F for 10 minutes.
7. Serve and enjoy.

Flavorful Chickpeas

Preparation time: 10 minutes

Cooking time: 10 minutes

Servings: 4

Nutritional Values (per Serving):

- Calories 155
- Fat 5.3 g
- Carbohydrates 22.8 g
- Sugar 0 g
- Protein 5.8 g
- Cholesterol 2 mg

Ingredients:

- 14 oz can chickpeas, drained and rinsed
- 1 tbsp Parmesan cheese, grated
- 1/8 tsp garlic powder
- 1 tbsp olive oil

- 1/8 tsp cayenne
- Pepper
- Salt

Directions:

1. Preheat the air fryer to 400 F.
2. Add all ingredients into the bowl and toss well.
3. Add chickpeas into the air fryer basket and cook for 10 minutes. Stir halfway through.
4. Serve and enjoy.

Sweet Potato Fries

Preparation time: 10 minutes

Cooking time: 20 minutes

Servings: 2

Nutritional Values (per Serving):

- Calories 95
- Fat 4.8 g
- Carbohydrates 12 g
- Sugar 3.7 g
- Protein 1.2 g
- Cholesterol 0 mg

Ingredients:

- 1 sweet potato, peeled and cut into fries shape
- 2 tsp olive oil
- 1/8 tsp cayenne
- 1/4 tsp chili powder

- Pepper
- Salt

Directions:

1. Preheat the air fryer to 400 F.
2. Spray air fryer basket with cooking spray.
3. Add all ingredients into the bowl and toss well.
4. Add sweet potato fries into the air fryer basket and cook for 20 minutes. Turn halfway through.
5. Serve and enjoy.

Healthy Pumpkin Seeds

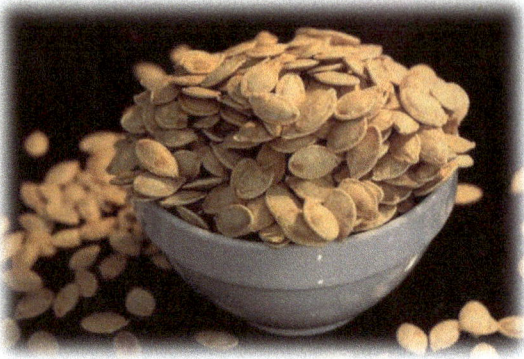

Preparation time: 10 minutes

Cooking time: 10 minutes

Servings: 8

Nutritional Values (per Serving):

- Calories 210
- Fat 17.6 g
- Carbohydrates 8.4 g
- Sugar 2.6 g
- Protein 8.5 g
- Cholesterol 0 mg

Ingredients:

- 2 cups pumpkin seeds
- 2 tbsp brown sugar
- 1 tsp vinegar
- 1 tbsp olive oil
- 1 tsp kosher salt

Directions:

1. Preheat the air fryer to 325 F.
2. Add all ingredients into the bowl and toss well.
3. Add pumpkin seeds into the air fryer basket and cook for 10 minutes. Stir halfway through.
4. Serve and enjoy.

Avocado and Almond Sweet Cream

Preparation time: 20 minutes

Cooking time: 0 minutes

Servings: 6

Nutritional Values (Per Serving):

- Calories 106
- Fat 3.4
- Fiber 0
- Carbs 2.4
- Protein 4

Ingredients:

- 2 avocados, peeled, pitted and mashed

- 1 cup coconut cream
- 2 tablespoons stevia
- 1 teaspoon almond extract
- ¾ cup stevia
- ¾ cup almonds, ground

Directions:

In a blender, combine the avocados with the cream and the other ingredients, pulse well, divide into cups and keep in the fridge for at least 20 minutes before serving.

Mint Rice Pudding

Preparation time: 10 minutes

Cooking time: 30 minutes

Servings: 4

Nutritional Values (Per Serving):

- Calories 200
- Fat 6.3
- Fiber 2
- Carbs 6.5
- Protein 8

Ingredients:

- ¼ cup stevia
- 2 cups cauliflower rice
- 2 cups coconut milk
- 2 tablespoons walnuts, chopped
- 1 tablespoon mint, chopped

- 1 teaspoon lime zest, grated
- ½ cup coconut cream

Directions:

1. In a pan, combine the cauliflower rice with the stevia, the coconut milk and the other ingredients, whisk, bring to a simmer and cook over medium-low heat for 30 minutes.
2. Divide the pudding into bowls and serve.

Walnuts and Coconut Cake

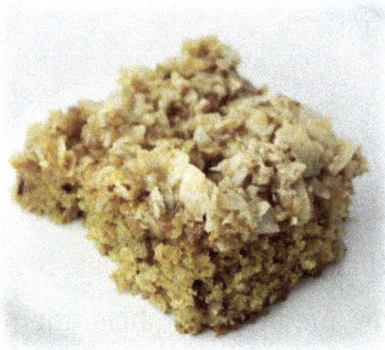

Preparation time: 10 minutes

Cooking time: 30 minutes

Servings: 8

Nutritional Values (Per Serving):

- Calories 200
- Fat 7.6
- Fiber 2.5
- Carbs 5.5
- Protein 4.5

Ingredients:

- 2 cups almond flour
- 2 teaspoons baking powder
- 1 cup avocado oil
- 1 cup coconut flesh, unsweetened and shredded
- 2 cups coconut milk
- 1 cup stevia
- 1 cup coconut cream
- 2 tablespoons walnuts, chopped
- 1 tablespoon lime juice
- 2 teaspoons vanilla extract
- Cooking spray

Directions:

1. In a bowl, mix the almond flour with the avocado oil, the coconut flesh, coconut milk and the other ingredients except the cooking spray and whisk well.
2. Pour the mix into a cake pan greased with the cooking spray, introduce in the oven and bake at 370 degrees F for 30 minutes.
3. Leave the cake to cool down, cut and serve!

Dates Cream

Preparation time: 10 minutes

Cooking time: 0 minutes

Servings: 2

Nutritional Values (Per Serving):

- Calories 192
- Fat 3.4
- Fiber 4.5
- Carbs 7.6
- Protein 3.5

Ingredients:

- 2 cups dates, chopped
- 1 cup coconut cream
- 2 tablespoons stevia
- 1 teaspoon vanilla extract

- 2 tablespoons water
- ½ teaspoon nutmeg, ground

Directions:

1. In a blender, combine the dates with the cream, the stevia and the other ingredients, pulse well, divide into cups and serve cold.

Chia Bowls

Preparation time: 5 minutes

Cooking time: 0 minutes

Servings: 2

Nutritional Values (Per Serving):

- Calories 182
- Fat 3.4
- Fiber 3.4
- Carbs 8.4
- Protein 3

Ingredients:

- 2 cups coconut milk, warm
- ½ cup coconut cream
- 1 cup cauliflower rice, steamed
- 2 tablespoons stevia

- 2 tablespoons chia seeds
- 1 teaspoon cinnamon powder

Directions:

1. In a bowl, combine the cream with the milk, the cauliflower rice and the other ingredients, whisk, well, leave aside for 5 minutes, divide into small bowls and serve cold.

Coconut Cream

Preparation time: 5 minutes

Cooking time: 0 minutes

Servings: 2

Nutritional Values (Per Serving):

- Calories 193
- Fat 5.4
- Fiber 3.4
- Carbs 7.6
- Protein 3

Ingredients:

- 2 cups coconut flesh, unsweetened shredded
- 3 tablespoons mint, chopped
- 2 cups coconut cream
- 2 tablespoons stevia
- ½ teaspoon cocoa powder

Directions:

1. In a blender, combine the coconut flesh with the mint, the cream and the other ingredients, pulse well, divide into cups and serve cold.

Watermelon and Rhubarb Cream

Preparation time: 10 minutes

Cooking time: 0 minutes

Servings: 2

Nutritional Values (Per Serving):

- Calories 122
- Fat 5.7
- Fiber 3.2
- Carbs 5.3
- Protein 0.4

Ingredients:

- 1 pound watermelon, peeled and chopped
- 1 cup rhubarb, chopped
- 1 teaspoon vanilla extract

- 1 cup coconut cream
- 1 teaspoon lime juice
- 2 teaspoons lime zest, grated

Directions:

1. In a blender, combine the watermelon with the rhubarb, the vanilla and the rest of the ingredients, pulse well, divide into cups and keep in the fridge before serving.

Rhubarb Stew

Preparation time: 10 minutes

Cooking time: 10 minutes

Servings: 4

Nutritional Values (Per Serving):

- Calories 122
- Fat 3.7
- Fiber 1.2
- Carbs 2.3
- Protein 0.4

Ingredients:

- 2 tablespoons stevia
- 1 cup water
- 1 teaspoon vanilla extract
- 1 teaspoon lemon zest, grated

- Juice of ½ lemon
- 2 cups rhubarb, roughly chopped

Directions:

1. Heat up a pan with the water over medium heat, add the stevia, the rhubarb and the other ingredients, toss, simmer for 10 minutes, divide into cups and serve cold.

Spicy Jalapeno Brussels sprouts

Preparation time: 5 minutes

Cooking time: 10 minutes

Servings: 4

Nutritions:

- Calories 91
- Fat 3.9g
- Carbohydrates 13.1g
- Sugar 3.7g
- Protein 4.2g
- Cholesterol 0mg

Ingredients:

- 1 lb Brussels sprouts
- 1 medium onion, chopped
- 1 tbsp olive oil
- 1 jalapeno pepper, seeded and chopped
- Pepper
- Salt

Directions:

1. Heat olive oil in a pan over medium heat.
2. Add onion and jalapeno in the pan and sauté until softened.
3. Add Brussels sprouts and stir until golden brown, about 10 minutes.
4. Season with pepper and salt.
5. Serve and enjoy.

Sage Pecan Cauliflower

Preparation time: 10 minutes

Cooking time: 30 minutes

Servings: 6

Nutritions:

- Calories 118
- Fat 8.6g
- Carbohydrates 9.9g
- Sugar 4.2g
- Protein 3.1g
- Cholesterol 0mg

Ingredients:

- 1 large cauliflower head, cut into florets
- 1/2 tsp dried thyme
- 1/2 tsp poultry seasoning
- 1/4 cup olive oil

- 2 garlic clove, minced
- 1/4 cup pecans, chopped
- 2 tbsp parsley, chopped
- 1/2 tsp ground sage
- 1/4 cup celery, chopped
- 1 onion, sliced
- 1/4 tsp black pepper
- 1 tsp sea salt

Directions:

1. Preheat the oven to 450 F/ 232 C.
2. Spray a baking tray with cooking spray and set aside.
3. In a large bowl, mix together cauliflower, thyme, poultry seasoning, olive oil, garlic, celery, sage, onions, pepper, and salt.
4. Spread mixture on a baking tray and roast in preheated oven for 15 minutes.
5. Add pecans and parsley and stir well. Roast for 10-15 minutes more.
6. Serve and enjoy.

Baked Cauliflower

Preparation time: 15 minutes

Cooking time: 40 minutes

Servings: 2

Nutritions:

- Calories 177
- Fat 15.6g
- Carbohydrates 11.5g
- Sugar 3.2g
- Protein 3.1g
- Cholesterol 0mg

Ingredients:

- 1/2 cauliflower head, cut into florets
- 2 tbsp olive oil

For seasoning:

- 1/2 tsp garlic powder
- 1/2 tsp ground cumin
- 1/2 tsp black pepper
- 1/2 tsp white pepper
- 1 tsp onion powder
- 1/4 tsp dried oregano
- 1/4 tsp dried basil
- 1/4 tsp dried thyme
- 1 tbsp ground cayenne pepper
- 2 tbsp ground paprika
- 2 tsp salt

Directions:

1. Preheat the oven to 400 F/ 200 C.
2. Spray a baking tray with cooking spray and set aside.
3. In a large bowl, mix together all seasoning ingredients.
4. Add oil and stir well. Add cauliflower to the bowl seasoning mixture and stir well to coat.
5. Spread the cauliflower florets on a baking tray and bake in preheated oven for 45 minutes.
6. Serve and enjoy.

Cabbage Cucumber Salad

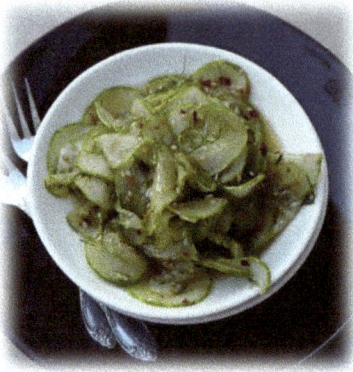

Preparation time: 20 minutes

Cooking time: 0 minute

Servings: 8

Nutritions:

- Calories 71
- Fat 5.4g
- Carbohydrates 5.9g
- Sugar 2.8g
- Protein 1.3g
- Cholesterol 0mg

Ingredients:

- 1/2 cabbage head, chopped
- 2 cucumbers, sliced
- 2 tbsp green onion, chopped
- 2 tbsp fresh dill, chopped
- 3 tbsp olive oil
- 1/2 lemon juice
- Pepper
- Salt

Directions:

1. Add cabbage to the large bowl. Season with 1 teaspoon of salt mix well and set aside.
2. Add cucumbers, green onions, and fresh dill. Mix well.
3. Add lemon juice, pepper, olive oil, and salt. Mix well.
4. Place salad bowl in refrigerator for 2 hours.
5. Serve chilled and enjoy.

Avocado Cucumber Soup

Preparation time: 40 minutes

Cooking time: 0 minute

Servings: 3

Nutritions:

- Calories 73
- Fat 3.7g
- Carbohydrates 9.2g
- Sugar 2.8g
- Protein 2.2g
- Cholesterol 0mg

Ingredients:

- 1 large cucumber, peeled and sliced
- ¾ cup water
- ¼ cup lemon juice
- 2 garlic cloves

- 6 green onion
- 2 avocados, pitted
- ½ tsp black pepper
- ½ tsp pink salt

Directions:

1. Add all ingredients into the blender and blend until smooth and creamy.
2. Place in refrigerator for 30 minutes.
3. Stir well and serve chilled.

Basil Tomato Soup

Preparation time: 5 minutes

Cooking time: 15 minutes

Servings: 6

Nutritions:

- Calories 30
- Fat 0g
- Carbohydrates 12.1g
- Sugar 9.6g
- Protein 1.3g
- Cholesterol 0mg

Ingredients:

- 28 oz can tomatoes
- ¼ cup basil pesto
- ¼ tsp dried basil leaves
- 1 tsp apple cider vinegar

- 2 tbsp erythritol
- ¼ tsp garlic powder
- ½ tsp onion powder
- 2 cups water
- 1 ½ tsp kosher salt

Directions:

1. Add tomatoes, garlic powder, onion powder, water, and salt in a saucepan.
2. Bring to boil over medium heat. Reduce heat and simmer for 2 minutes.
3. Remove saucepan from heat and puree the soup using a blender until smooth.
4. Stir in pesto, dried basil, vinegar, and erythritol.
5. Stir well and serve warm.

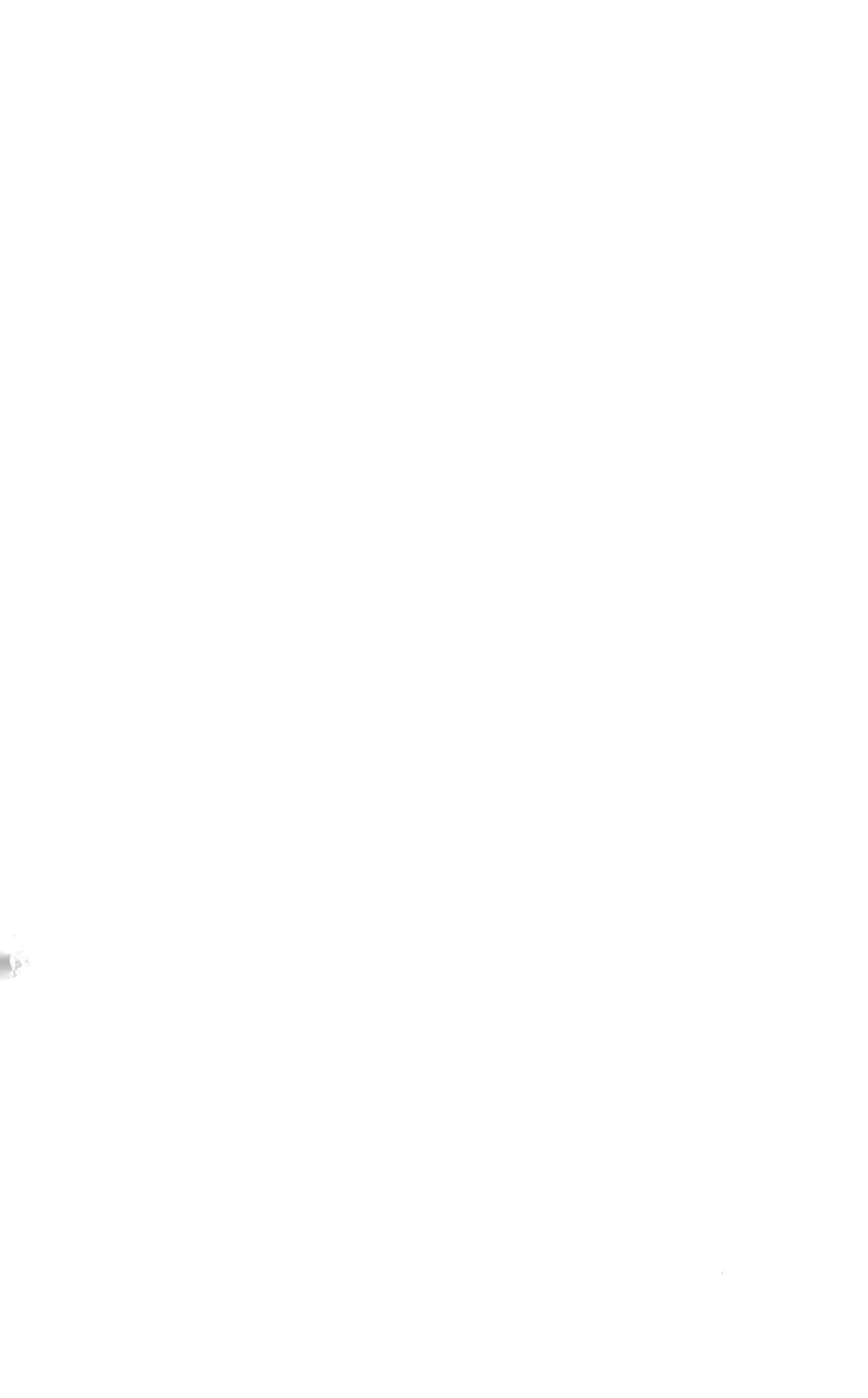

www.ingramcontent.com/pod-product-compliance
Lightning Source LLC
Chambersburg PA
CBHW050746030426
42336CB00012B/1681